UNDERSTANDING CANINE DIABETES

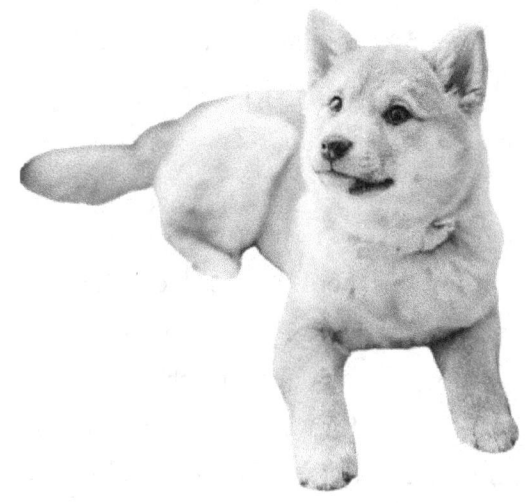

A Comprehensive Guide to Diagnosis, Treatment, and Care

Jennie Jonas

Understanding Canine Cancer: A Comprehensive Guide to Diagnosis, Treatment, and Care

Copyright © 2024 [Jennie Jonas]. All rights reserved.

No part of this publication may be reproduced, distributed, or transmitted in any form or by any means, including photocopying, recording, or other electronic or mechanical methods, without the prior written permission of the publisher, except in the case of brief quotations embodied in critical reviews and certain other noncommercial uses permitted by copyright law.

This book is a work of nonfiction. The information provided within this book is based on the author's research, knowledge, and experiences. While the author has made every effort to ensure the accuracy and completeness of the information contained within this book, it is not intended as a substitute for professional veterinary advice. Always consult with a qualified veterinarian for medical advice and treatment tailored to your pet's specific needs.

First Edition, 2024

Table Of Contents

INTRODUCTION 5
Chapter 01 7
What is Canine Diabetes? 7
Chapter 02 17
Common Symptoms of Diabetes in Dogs 17
Chapter 03 31
Diagnosing Diabetes in Dogs 31
Chapter 04 43
Treatment Options for Canine Diabetes 43
Chapter 05 49
Making Treatment Decisions for Your Dog 49
Chapter 06 55
Managing Side Effects of Diabetes Treatment . 55
Chapter 07 61
Nutrition and Diet for Dogs with Diabetes 61
Chapter 08 67
Dietary Recommendations for Diabetic Dogs .. 67
Chapter 09 71
Recipes for Diabetic Dogs 71
Chapter 10 85
Additional Tips for Managing Diabetes in Dogs .. 85
Chapter 11 89
Alternative Therapies for Canine Diabetes 89
Chapter 12 95
Emotional Support for You and Your Family 95
Conclusion 101

Note

Introduction

The journey of caring for a diabetic dog is both a challenging and rewarding one that I never expected to embark on myself. It all began with subtle changes in my dog's behavior, he was drinking more water than usual, urinating frequently, and seemed to be losing weight despite his normal diet. Concerned, I took him to the vet, where a blood test confirmed what I had feared: diabetes!

At first, the diagnosis felt overwhelming. I was flooded with questions. What caused this? How would we manage it? Would my dog's quality of life suffer? While I received excellent guidance from my veterinarian, I realized that many pet owners might not have the same level of support or access to information. This experience fueled my determination to learn everything I could about canine diabetes and eventually led me to write this book.

This guide not only breaks down the medical side of diabetes but also offers practical advice on managing day-to-day life with a diabetic dog. This book is the result of that journey, a resource built to help you understand what diabetes means for your dog, how to manage it effectively, and most importantly, how to ensure your dog continues to live a happy, fulfilling life. Understanding the nuances of diabetes, recognizing the signs early, and working closely with your veterinarian can make a significant difference in how well the condition is managed and how healthy and happy your dog remains.

This book will walk you through the essentials of diabetes care, offering practical tips on everything from insulin administration to dietary recommendations, and providing emotional support along the way. Your journey, like mine, will be filled with learning, adapting, and ultimately, discovering how resilient and strong both you and your dog can be.

Chapter 01

What is Canine Diabetes?

Diabetes in dogs is a chronic condition that affects the body's ability to regulate glucose, a vital source of energy. When a dog consumes food, their body breaks down carbohydrates into glucose, which enters the bloodstream. Normally, insulin, a hormone produced by the pancreas, allows glucose to enter cells and be used for energy. In diabetic dogs, this process is disrupted, either the pancreas does not produce enough insulin, or the body's cells cannot effectively use the insulin it produces. This leads to elevated blood sugar levels, a condition called hyperglycemia, which can cause significant health problems if left untreated.

Diabetes is a lifelong condition, but with proper management, including insulin therapy, diet adjustments, and regular monitoring, dogs can live healthy, active lives. Understanding the basics of how diabetes works is the first step in managing your dog's condition effectively.

How Diabetes Affects a Dog's Body

The absence or inefficiency of insulin means that glucose remains in the bloodstream instead of being used by the cells for energy. The body starts breaking down fat and muscle for fuel, leading to weight loss and other complications. Meanwhile, the excess glucose in the blood is excreted through urine, which leads to increased urination and thirst as the body tries to flush out the excess sugar. Over time, this chronic high blood sugar can lead to a range of health issues, including:

Organ Damage: Prolonged high blood sugar can damage vital organs, including the kidneys, liver, and heart. This can lead to conditions like diabetic nephropathy (kidney damage).

Vision Problems: High glucose levels can cause cataracts in dogs, leading to cloudy vision or even blindness.

Nerve Damage: In some cases, diabetes can cause neuropathy, or nerve damage, which may affect coordination or cause pain.

In dogs, the body may also begin breaking down fat and muscle tissue for energy, leading to unintended weight loss despite a normal or increased appetite. This is because, without insulin, the cells are effectively "starved" for energy, even though there's plenty of glucose in the blood.

1. Types of Diabetes in Dogs

Dogs, like humans, can suffer from two main types of diabetes:

A. Type 1 Diabetes (Insulin-Dependent Diabetes Mellitus)

Description: Type 1 diabetes is the most common form in dogs and is characterized by the pancreas's inability to produce enough insulin. In this case, insulin therapy is essential to maintain proper blood sugar levels.

Cause: This form of diabetes is usually caused by the immune system attacking and destroying the insulin-producing cells in the pancreas, making the dog reliant on external insulin for life.

Management: Dogs with Type 1 diabetes require daily insulin injections to help regulate blood sugar, alongside careful management of their diet and exercise routine.

B. Type 2 Diabetes (Non-Insulin-Dependent Diabetes)

Description: Type 2 diabetes, though rare in dogs, involves insulin resistance—where the dog's body can produce insulin, but the cells do not respond to it properly. This form is more common in overweight or obese dogs.

Cause: Type 2 diabetes is often linked to factors like poor diet and lack of exercise, leading to obesity, which increases the risk of insulin resistance.

Management: While diet, weight loss, and lifestyle changes can sometimes reduce the severity of Type 2 diabetes, some dogs will still require insulin injections for proper glucose management.

C. Gestational Diabetes

Another less common form of diabetes is gestational diabetes, which occurs in pregnant female dogs due to hormonal changes. This form of diabetes is typically temporary and resolves after the pregnancy, though it can sometimes lead to long-term insulin issues if not properly managed.

Recognizing which type of diabetes your dog has will influence the course of treatment. Your veterinarian will determine the appropriate approach based on diagnostic tests, including blood glucose levels and clinical symptoms.

2. Causes and Risk Factors

The exact cause of diabetes in dogs can vary, but several risk factors have been identified that can make certain dogs more prone to developing the condition:

A. Genetics and Breed Predisposition

Genetics plays a significant role in the development of diabetes in dogs. Some breeds are more prone to developing diabetes due to hereditary factors that affect their pancreas or insulin production.

Breeds at Higher Risk: Certain dog breeds have a higher genetic predisposition to diabetes. These include:
- *Beagles*
- *Miniature Schnauzers*
- *Poodles (especially Miniature and Toy Poodles)*

- Samoyeds

- Dachshunds

- Keeshonds

- Australian Terriers

These breeds are more likely to develop Type 1 diabetes, where the pancreas is unable to produce adequate insulin due to autoimmune damage. Owners of these breeds should be especially vigilant for early signs of diabetes.

B. Age

Age is another key risk factor for diabetes in dogs. Most cases of canine diabetes are diagnosed in middle-aged to older dogs, typically between the ages of 6 and 9 years. Older dogs are at an increased risk because their bodies are more likely to experience a decline in insulin production or develop insulin resistance. Younger dogs are less commonly affected but can still develop diabetes, particularly if they have a genetic predisposition or certain medical conditions.

C. Obesity

Obesity is a significant risk factor for diabetes, especially Type 2 diabetes, where insulin resistance plays a major role. Overweight dogs are more likely to develop insulin resistance, where the body produces insulin but the cells fail to respond effectively. This leads to elevated blood sugar levels, which can eventually exhaust the pancreas, causing diabetes. Fat cells release certain hormones and substances that can interfere with insulin's effectiveness, further contributing to the development of the disease. Maintaining a healthy weight through a balanced diet and regular exercise is crucial in reducing a dog's risk of diabetes, particularly for breeds prone to obesity.

D. Gender

Female dogs, especially those that are not spayed, are at a higher risk of developing diabetes compared to male dogs. They are twice as likely to develop diabetes, primarily due to hormonal influences, especially related to progesterone and estrogen, which can affect insulin regulation. Intact females may experience fluctuating hormone levels during their reproductive cycles, which can interfere with insulin regulation and increase the likelihood of diabetes. Spaying a female dog reduces the risk of diabetes, as it helps stabilize hormone levels and reduces the strain on the pancreas.

E. Autoimmune Disease

In Type 1 diabetes, the immune system attacks the cells in the pancreas responsible for insulin production. This autoimmune response is believed to be a key cause of insulin-dependent diabetes.

F. Pancreatitis

Diseases that affect the pancreas can lead to diabetes, especially if they damage the insulin-producing beta cells. Chronic pancreatitis (inflammation of the pancreas) is a major contributor to diabetes in dogs. Repeated bouts of pancreatitis can damage the pancreas over time, reducing its ability to produce insulin. In other words dogs with a history of pancreatitis are at higher risk of developing diabetes later in life. Pancreatic insufficiency or pancreatic tumors can also affect insulin production and regulation, leading to the development of diabetes.

G. Certain Medications

Prolonged use of medications like steroids can contribute to diabetes in dogs by affecting the pancreas and altering the body's ability to regulate glucose. If your dog has been on long-term medication, they may be at higher risk for diabetes.

Understanding the causes and risk factors associated with diabetes in dogs can help in both preventing the condition and managing it more effectively when it does arise. Early detection and intervention can make a significant difference in the long-term health and well-being of your dog.

Note

Chapter 02

Common Symptoms of Diabetes in Dogs

Recognizing the symptoms of diabetes in dogs is key to ensuring early diagnosis and treatment. If your dog is exhibiting any of these signs, especially increased thirst, frequent urination, or unexplained weight loss—it's important to visit a veterinarian for an evaluation. Early detection can make a significant difference in managing the disease and preventing serious complications like diabetic ketoacidosis, cataracts, or organ damage. With proper treatment, including insulin therapy and dietary management, diabetic dogs can lead long, healthy lives.

1. Recognizing the Signs of Diabetes

Early recognition of diabetes in dogs is crucial for effective management and treatment. While the symptoms may vary from dog to dog, there are several common signs that you should be aware of. These symptoms often appear gradually, so it's essential to monitor your dog closely if you suspect they may be developing diabetes. The most common signs include:

A. Increased Thirst (Polydipsia)

One of the earliest and most noticeable signs of diabetes in dogs is excessive thirst. Diabetic dogs often drink more water than usual because the high levels of glucose in their blood pull water from their tissues, leading to dehydration. As a result, the dog feels persistently thirsty and drinks large amounts of water.

What to Look For: You may notice your dog drinking from their water bowl more frequently or even seeking out unusual sources of water, like faucets or puddles. This increased thirst may be especially noticeable in dogs that were previously moderate drinkers.

B. Increased Urination (Polyuria)

Increased urination, or polyuria, often accompanies excessive thirst. As the body attempts to get rid of excess glucose by flushing it out through the kidneys, more urine is produced. This leads to frequent urination and larger volumes of urine each time.

What to Look For: You might observe that your dog is asking to go outside more often than usual, especially during the night, or is having accidents indoors. The volume of urine passed is typically much higher than normal. The body is trying to eliminate excess glucose through urine, which leads to this increased urination.

C. Weight Loss Despite a Normal or Increased Appetite

A common symptom of diabetes in dogs is unexplained weight loss, even if the dog is eating more than usual. Since the body cannot properly use glucose for energy, it begins breaking down fat and muscle for fuel, leading to weight loss.

What to Look For: You may notice your dog becoming thinner or losing muscle mass, particularly along the spine or hips, despite having a healthy or increased appetite.

D. Fatigue and Lethargy

As diabetes progresses, affected dogs may become lethargic, tired and less energetic. This lack of energy occurs because the body cannot convert glucose into usable energy, leaving your dog feeling weak and fatigued, even after periods of rest.

What to Look For: Your dog may seem less active, tire more easily during play or walks, and prefer to rest more often. This lethargy can appear suddenly or gradually worsen over time.

E. Cloudy Eyes (Cataracts)
One of the long-term complications of diabetes in dogs is the development of cataracts, which can cause the eyes to appear cloudy. High blood sugar levels can lead to changes in the lens of the eye, causing it to become opaque.

What to Look For: Cloudiness or a bluish tint in your dog's eyes, as well as changes in their vision. Dogs may bump into objects or appear disoriented in familiar surroundings. This symptom is particularly common in dogs with advanced diabetes and it (Cataracts) can progress quickly and may lead to blindness if not treated.

F. Increased Hunger (Polyphagia)
Diabetic dogs often experience increased appetite or ravenous hunger. This is because their bodies are unable to use the glucose from food for energy, so they constantly feel hungry, even though they are eating plenty.

What to Look For: Your dog may seem hungrier than usual, begging for food more often, or showing aggressive behavior around meals. However, despite the increased food intake, weight loss may still occur.

G. Sweet or Fruity-Smelling Breath

Diabetic dogs sometimes develop sweet or fruity-smelling breath due to a condition called ketoacidosis, which occurs when the body begins breaking down fat for energy in the absence of glucose. This is a serious complication of unmanaged diabetes and can be life-threatening if not addressed promptly.

What to Look For: A noticeable change in the smell of your dog's breath, along with other symptoms of illness, such as vomiting, lethargy, and dehydration. Ketoacidosis is a medical emergency that requires immediate veterinary attention.

H. Urinary Tract Infections (UTIs)

High blood sugar levels create an ideal environment for bacteria to thrive, leading to urinary tract infections (UTIs). Diabetic dogs may develop frequent UTIs because the excess sugar in their urine can foster bacterial growth in the urinary tract.

What to Look For: Symptoms of a UTI include difficulty urinating, straining, frequent attempts to urinate with little output, blood in the urine, or discomfort when urinating. If your dog has recurring UTIs, this may be a sign of underlying diabetes.

I. Dehydration

Since diabetic dogs lose more water through frequent urination, they may become **dehydrated** despite drinking large amounts of water.

What to Look For: Signs of dehydration include dry gums, sunken eyes, lethargy, and loss of skin elasticity (when you pinch the skin, it takes longer to return to its normal position). Dehydration is a serious condition and should be addressed quickly to prevent further health complications.

J. Poor Coat Condition and Skin Issues

Dogs with uncontrolled diabetes may develop a poor coat condition and experience skin problems. This can result from malnutrition or the body's inability to properly metabolize nutrients.

What to Look For: A dull, dry coat or hair loss, along with flaky or irritated skin. Diabetic dogs may also be more prone to infections or take longer to heal from wounds or skin irritations.

Recognizing the symptoms of diabetes in dogs is key to ensuring early diagnosis and treatment. If your dog is exhibiting any of these signs, especially increased thirst, frequent urination, or unexplained weight loss, it's important to visit a veterinarian for an evaluation. Early detection can make a significant difference in managing the disease and preventing serious complications like diabetic ketoacidosis, cataracts, or organ damage. With proper treatment, including insulin therapy and dietary management, diabetic dogs can lead long, healthy lives.

2. **Differentiating Diabetes from Other Conditions**

While the symptoms of diabetes in dogs can seem clear, they are sometimes mistaken for other medical conditions. Recognizing the subtle differences between diabetes and other diseases with similar symptoms is key to getting the right diagnosis and treatment. Here's how they compare:

A. Increased Thirst and Urination (Polydipsia and Polyuria): Diabetes vs. Kidney Disease

Diabetes Mellitus: Excessive thirst and urination are common in both diabetes and kidney disease. In diabetes, these symptoms are driven by the body's attempt to flush out excess glucose through urine. The kidneys work harder, and water is drawn out, leading to dehydration and polydipsia (excessive thirst). These symptoms are usually accompanied by other signs like weight loss and increased hunger.

Kidney Disease: With kidney disease, the kidneys are unable to retain water properly, leading to increased urination and subsequent thirst. However, Chronic kidney disease (CKD) often leads to additional symptoms, such as vomiting, loss of appetite, bad breath, and ulcers in the mouth. Blood tests showing elevated kidney markers, such as creatinine and urea, help differentiate CKD from diabetes.

B. Weight Loss Despite Normal or Increased Appetite: Diabetes vs. Hyperthyroidism and other diseases

Unexplained weight loss can be a hallmark of diabetes, but it can also occur with other conditions:

Cushing's Disease: Dogs with Cushing's disease (hyperadrenocorticism) also exhibit increased hunger, but the cause is different—an overproduction of cortisol, a stress hormone. However, these dogs tend to gain weight, have a pot-bellied appearance, and show thinning of the skin. A diagnostic test for cortisol levels can help distinguish Cushing's from diabetes.

Diabetes Mellitus: In diabetes, weight loss occurs because the body is unable to use glucose for energy, so it breaks down fat and muscle instead. This is often accompanied by increased hunger (polyphagia) and thirst.

Hyperthyroidism: Although rare in dogs (more common in cats), hyperthyroidism can cause weight loss despite a normal or increased appetite. Dogs with hyperthyroidism may also show signs of hyperactivity, increased heart rate, and heat intolerance. Blood tests measuring thyroid hormone levels can confirm hyperthyroidism.

Exocrine Pancreatic Insufficiency (EPI): EPI is a condition in which the pancreas does not produce enough digestive enzymes, leading to weight loss and increased appetite. Dogs with EPI often have loose, greasy stools. A fecal test or enzyme blood test helps differentiate EPI from diabetes.

Cancer: Certain cancers, particularly those affecting the gastrointestinal tract or organs involved in metabolism, can cause weight loss despite a normal or increased appetite. Cancer is usually associated with other symptoms, such as lethargy, vomiting, or abnormal masses.

Urinary Tract Infections (UTIs): While UTIs can cause frequent urination, they are typically associated with discomfort during urination, blood in the urine, or straining. UTIs do not usually cause increased thirst or weight loss, helping distinguish them from diabetes.

B. Lethargy and Fatigue:

Fatigue and reduced energy levels can be seen in many diseases, including diabetes. Here's how to differentiate them:

Diabetes Mellitus: Fatigue in diabetic dogs is due to the lack of usable energy from glucose. It is typically accompanied by other classic signs, such as increased thirst and urination, weight loss, and changes in appetite.

Hypothyroidism: Hypothyroidism, a condition in which the thyroid gland is underactive, can cause lethargy and weight gain, along with dry skin and a dull coat. This is the opposite of diabetes, where dogs typically lose weight. Blood tests measuring thyroid hormone levels can confirm hypothyroidism.

Heart Disease: Fatigue in heart disease is often associated with coughing, difficulty breathing, or exercise intolerance. Dogs with heart disease may experience fluid accumulation, which leads to a swollen abdomen and laboured breathing, helping differentiate it from diabetes.

Anaemia: Anaemia, or a low red blood cell count, can cause weakness and lethargy. Unlike diabetes, anemia is often associated with pale gums, rapid breathing, and sometimes bloody stools or vomiting. Blood tests measuring red blood cell counts can distinguish anemia from diabetes.

C. Cataracts: Diabetes vs. Eye Diseases

Cataracts are a well-known complication of diabetes, but other conditions can also affect your dog's vision:

Diabetes Mellitus: Cataracts in diabetic dogs develop rapidly due to high blood sugar levels, which cause changes in the lens of the eye. Diabetic cataracts often occur in combination with other diabetes symptoms like increased thirst, urination, and weight loss.

Genetic Cataracts: Some breeds are prone to hereditary cataracts that are unrelated to diabetes. These cataracts usually develop slowly and do not coincide with systemic symptoms like excessive thirst or urination.

Progressive Retinal Atrophy (PRA): PRA is a genetic condition that causes gradual vision loss due to degeneration of the retina. Unlike cataracts, PRA does not cause the lens to become cloudy and is not related to diabetes. Dogs with PRA typically have night blindness as an early sign.

Glaucoma: Glaucoma, a condition characterized by increased pressure in the eye, can lead to vision problems and pain. Symptoms include redness, squinting, and a cloudy cornea. Unlike cataracts from diabetes, glaucoma is typically painful and causes eye enlargement.

D. Sweet-Smelling Breath

While sweet-smelling or fruity breath is a hallmark of diabetic ketoacidosis (DKA), other conditions can cause bad breath:

Diabetes Mellitus: In diabetic ketoacidosis, the body produces ketones due to the lack of glucose for energy, resulting in fruity-smelling breath. This is a medical emergency and usually occurs in conjunction with vomiting, lethargy, and dehydration.

Kidney Disease: Dogs with kidney disease may have bad breath due to the buildup of toxins in the blood (uremia), but the smell is often described as "ammonia-like" rather than fruity. Kidney disease is also associated with increased thirst and urination, making it easy to confuse with diabetes.

Dental Disease: Poor oral hygiene or dental infections can lead to bad breath, but it is usually foul-smelling rather than sweet. Dental disease typically does not cause systemic symptoms like increased thirst or weight loss.

While many of the symptoms of diabetes in dogs can overlap with other conditions, understanding the context in which they occur, and working closely with your veterinarian to get accurate tests, is critical to ensuring your dog receives the proper treatment. By recognizing the key signs of diabetes early and differentiating it from other health problems, you can take proactive steps to manage your dog's condition and maintain their well-being.

Chapter 03

Diagnosing Diabetes in Dogs

Diagnosing diabetes in dogs involves a comprehensive evaluation that includes a physical examination, medical history, and specific laboratory tests. Early detection is crucial for effective management of the disease, which can help prevent complications and improve the quality of life for your furry friend. Here's a detailed look at the steps involved in diagnosing diabetes in dogs:

1. Veterinary Consultation

The first step in diagnosing diabetes is to consult your veterinarian. They will begin by taking a thorough medical history, including:

Symptoms: Discuss any signs your dog has been exhibiting, such as increased thirst (polydipsia), frequent urination (polyuria), unexplained weight loss, increased appetite, lethargy, or changes in coat condition.

Diet and Lifestyle: Provide information about your dog's diet, exercise routine, and any recent changes in behavior or health.

Previous Medical Conditions: Inform the veterinarian about any existing health issues, medications, or treatments your dog has received.

2. Physical Examination

During the physical examination, the veterinarian will assess your dog's overall health and look for specific signs that could indicate diabetes, including:

Body Condition: Evaluating your dog's weight and muscle condition to determine if they are underweight or overweight.

Hydration Levels: Checking for signs of dehydration, such as dry gums or sunken eyes.

Skin and Coat: Examining the skin and coat for any abnormalities, such as dryness or excessive shedding.

Eye Health: Assessing for signs of cataracts or other eye issues that could indicate diabetes.

Abdominal Examination: Palpating the abdomen to check for any abnormalities or signs of organ enlargement.

3. Laboratory Tests

Once the veterinarian suspects diabetes, they will recommend several laboratory tests to confirm the diagnosis:

A. Blood Tests:

- ***Blood Glucose Level:*** A blood sample is taken, usually from a vein in the dog's leg, to measure the concentration of glucose in the bloodstream. In healthy dogs, blood glucose levels are usually between 70-150 mg/dL. Levels above this range, especially persistent hyperglycemia, may indicate diabetes.

- ***Fructosamine Test:*** This test measures the average blood glucose levels over the previous two to three weeks. A blood sample is taken and analyzed for fructosamine, which is formed when glucose binds to proteins in the blood. Elevated fructosamine levels can indicate chronic hyperglycemia, helping to confirm a diabetes diagnosis and assess long-term glucose control. This test is particularly useful in differentiating stress-related increases in blood sugar (common during veterinary visits) from true diabetes.

B. Urinalysis:

Urinalysis is a key diagnostic tool that helps evaluate kidney function and the presence of glucose or ketones in the urine. The following components are typically assessed:

- ***Glucose in Urine:*** A urine sample is tested for the presence of glucose. In healthy dogs, there should be no glucose in the urine. A urine sample is collected (either by free catch or cystocentesis) and tested using a dipstick or laboratory analysis. The presence of glucose in urine indicates hyperglycemia, often associated with diabetes. In diabetic dogs, excess glucose that the body cannot process will spill over into the urine.

- ***Ketones in Urine:*** The presence of ketones in the urine may indicate diabetic ketoacidosis (DKA), a serious condition requiring immediate veterinary attention and can cause severe damage if poorly managed. This test can detect ketones, which are produced when the body breaks down fat for energy instead of glucose. Your veterinarian will collect a urine sample using a dipstick and test it for high glucose levels and the presence of ketones. The presence of ketones can indicate a more advanced stage of diabetes or diabetic ketoacidosis (DKA).

- ***Urinary Tract Infections:*** The urinalysis will also check for signs of infection, such as bacteria or white blood cells, which are common in diabetic dogs. Urine is cultured to detect the presence of bacteria.

C. Additional Diagnostic Tests

In some cases, additional diagnostic tests may be performed to rule out other conditions or complications:

Complete Blood Count (CBC): This test evaluates your dog's overall health and can identify underlying infections, anemia, or other issues. A blood sample is taken and analyzed for red and white blood cells and platelets. Abnormalities in blood cell counts may indicate concurrent health issues that require attention. This test helps rule out other illnesses that may present similar symptoms or identify complications associated with diabetes.

Biochemical Profile: A biochemical panel assesses organ function and checks for other metabolic disorders that may be contributing to your dog's symptoms. A blood sample is analyzed for various enzymes and substances produced by the liver, kidneys, and other organs. Results can reveal underlying conditions affecting diabetes management, such as liver or kidney disease.

Abdominal Ultrasound: In rare cases, imaging techniques like X-rays or ultrasound may be used to check for underlying conditions that could contribute to diabetes, such as pancreatitis or tumors affecting the pancreas and other abdominal organs for abnormalities that could affect diabetes management. These tests are not usually necessary for diagnosing diabetes but may be recommended if your dog has other unexplained symptoms or health issues.

D. Diagnosis Confirmation

Once all test results are available, the veterinarian will analyze the findings to confirm a diabetes diagnosis. If diabetes is diagnosed, the veterinarian will discuss the type of diabetes (typically Type 1 in dogs) and the best management plan tailored to your dog's needs.

E. Developing a Treatment Plan

After diagnosing diabetes, the veterinarian will work with you to create a comprehensive treatment plan that may include:

- ***Insulin Therapy:*** Most diabetic dogs require insulin injections to help regulate blood glucose levels.
- ***Dietary Changes:*** A special diet designed for diabetic dogs can help manage blood sugar levels.
- ***Regular Monitoring:*** Owners will be advised on how to monitor their dog's blood glucose levels at home and may need to schedule regular veterinary

check-ups to assess treatment effectiveness and make any necessary adjustments.

Diagnosing diabetes in dogs requires a combination of clinical evaluation and laboratory testing. By recognizing the signs and seeking veterinary care early, you can ensure timely diagnosis and appropriate management of your dog's condition. With proper treatment, diabetic dogs can lead healthy and fulfilling lives, and understanding the diagnosis process can help you be proactive in your pet's care.

4. Understanding Blood Sugar Levels

Monitoring your dog's blood sugar levels is critical to managing diabetes effectively. Understanding what these levels mean and how they fluctuate throughout the day will help you make informed decisions about insulin dosages, diet, and overall care.

A. Blood Glucose Ranges in Dogs

Normal Blood Sugar Levels: In healthy dogs, normal blood glucose levels typically range between 70 and 140 mg/dL. This range may vary slightly based on your veterinarian's guidelines.

Hyperglycemia (High Blood Sugar): Blood glucose levels above 200 mg/dL typically indicate hyperglycemia, which is a sign of poorly controlled diabetes. Consistently high blood sugar can lead to complications such as cataracts, neuropathy, and diabetic ketoacidosis (DKA).

Hypoglycemia (Low Blood Sugar): Blood sugar levels below 70 mg/dL are considered dangerously low. Hypoglycemia can cause weakness, disorientation, seizures, and even death if left untreated. It's essential to prevent hypoglycemia, particularly when administering insulin.

B. Importance of Consistent Monitoring

Keeping your dog's blood sugar within the target range is critical for preventing long-term complications. Regular monitoring helps ensure your dog's insulin dosage is correct and allows you to make dietary adjustments if necessary. Blood glucose levels can be affected by factors like:

- *Diet and Meal Timing*
- *Exercise*
- *Stress and Illness*
- *Insulin Dosage*

C. Using a Glucometer at Home

Many pet owners choose to monitor their dog's blood glucose levels at home using a handheld glucometer. This device measures blood glucose through a small drop of blood, usually collected from the ear or paw pad.

Benefits: Home monitoring provides real-time information on your dog's blood sugar, helping you adjust insulin dosages as needed. It also reduces the stress of frequent trips to the vet.

Procedure: Your veterinarian can show you how to safely and accurately use a glucometer, including how to obtain a blood sample and interpret the results.

5. Monitoring Your Dog's Condition

Managing diabetes is a lifelong commitment, and ongoing monitoring of your dog's condition is essential for long-term health. Here are some strategies for effective monitoring:

A. Regular Veterinary Visits

Frequency: Dogs with diabetes should see the veterinarian regularly, typically every 3 to 6 months. During these visits, your vet will evaluate your dog's overall health, perform blood tests to check glucose control, and adjust treatment as necessary.

Purpose: These appointments provide an opportunity to assess how well your dog's diabetes is being managed and to identify any early signs of complications, such as cataracts, kidney disease, or neuropathy.

B. Blood Glucose Curves

What It Is: A blood glucose curve involves taking blood sugar measurements at regular intervals throughout the day, usually every 2 hours. This allows your veterinarian to assess how well your dog's insulin is working and to adjust dosages as needed.

How It Helps: A glucose curve provides insight into your dog's blood sugar patterns, showing how glucose levels fluctuate in response to meals, insulin, and daily activity.

C. Monitoring for Symptoms

While regular blood glucose checks are essential, it's also important to monitor your dog's behavior and general health. Keep an eye out for changes in:

Appetite and Thirst: Increased hunger or thirst may indicate that your dog's blood sugar levels are not well controlled.

Urination: An increase in urination frequency may signal high blood sugar levels.

Energy Levels: If your dog seems unusually tired or lethargic, it could be a sign of high or low blood sugar.

Weight: Sudden or unexplained weight changes can indicate issues with diabetes management.

D. Keeping a Log

Why It's Important: Maintaining a detailed log of your dog's blood glucose levels, insulin dosages, food intake, and any symptoms helps you and your veterinarian track progress and make informed decisions about treatment.

What to Include: Record blood glucose readings, meal times, insulin administration times and doses, and any unusual behavior or symptoms. This information can be invaluable when adjusting treatment plans.

Accurate diagnosis and vigilant monitoring are the cornerstones of effective diabetes management in dogs. By understanding how to interpret blood sugar levels, performing regular tests, and keeping a close eye on your dog's overall health, you can ensure that your pet lives a comfortable, happy life despite their condition. Working closely with your veterinarian and using the tools available to monitor your dog's condition will empower you to make the best decisions for their care.

Note

Chapter 04

Treatment Options for Canine Diabetes

Managing diabetes in dogs requires a multifaceted approach that may involve insulin therapy, oral medications, and non-medication strategies. Each dog is unique, and treatment plans should be tailored to the individual pet based on their specific needs, lifestyle, and response to therapy.

1. INSULIN THERAPY

Insulin therapy is often the cornerstone of diabetes management for dogs, particularly for those diagnosed with Type 1 diabetes. Insulin is a hormone that helps regulate blood glucose levels by facilitating the uptake of glucose into the cells. Here's a closer look at insulin therapy:

A. Types of Insulin

- ***Short-Acting Insulin:*** This type provides quick control over blood glucose levels and is typically used during emergencies or for managing postprandial (after meals) glucose spikes.

- ***Intermediate-Acting Insulin:*** This insulin lasts longer than short-acting types and is often used for daily management. It helps maintain stable blood glucose levels throughout the day.

- ***Long-Acting Insulin:*** This type provides a more prolonged effect and is sometimes used in dogs that require less frequent dosing.

B. Administration

Injection Technique: Insulin is usually administered via subcutaneous injections (under the skin). It is crucial to rotate injection sites to prevent lipodystrophy and ensure proper absorption.

Dosage: Your veterinarian will determine the appropriate dosage based on your dog's weight, blood glucose levels, and overall health. Dosage adjustments may be necessary based on monitoring results.

C. Monitoring

Blood Glucose Monitoring: Regular blood glucose testing is essential to determine the effectiveness of insulin therapy and make necessary adjustments.

Signs of Hypoglycemia: Be vigilant for signs of low blood sugar, such as weakness, confusion, or seizures, especially after insulin administration.

D. Benefits and Challenges

Benefits: Insulin therapy effectively helps manage blood glucose levels, reduces the risk of diabetes-related complications, and improves your dog's quality of life.

Challenges: Proper administration and consistent monitoring can be demanding. Owners must be diligent in maintaining schedules and adjusting dosages as needed.

2. **ORAL MEDICATIONS**

While insulin therapy is the most common treatment for canine diabetes, certain dogs may benefit from oral medications. These medications are typically used in conjunction with dietary changes and monitoring.

A. Types of Oral Medications

Glipizide: This sulfonylurea medication stimulates the pancreas to produce more insulin. It is generally less effective in dogs than in humans but may be helpful for some dogs with Type 2 diabetes.

Metformin: Often used in human diabetes management, metformin helps improve insulin sensitivity and decrease glucose production by the liver. Its use in dogs is less common and should be evaluated on a case-by-case basis.

B. Considerations

Not Suitable for All Dogs: Oral medications are not universally effective in dogs, and many may still require insulin therapy. It's essential to work closely with your veterinarian to determine the best approach.

Monitoring: Regular blood glucose monitoring remains critical to assess the effectiveness of any oral medications and make necessary adjustments.

3. Non-Medication Approaches

In addition to insulin and oral medications, various non-medication approaches can support the management of canine diabetes. These strategies focus on lifestyle and dietary modifications that can help regulate blood sugar levels.

A. Dietary Management

Specialized Diets: Consult with your veterinarian to choose a high-fiber, low-glycemic diet designed specifically for diabetic dogs. These diets help stabilize blood glucose levels by slowing the absorption of glucose from the gastrointestinal tract.

Consistent Feeding Schedule: Feeding your dog at the same time each day helps regulate insulin levels and blood sugar. Avoid sudden changes in diet, as they can lead to fluctuations in glucose levels.

B. Weight Management

Maintaining a Healthy Weight: Obesity can worsen insulin resistance and complicate diabetes management. Work with your veterinarian to develop a weight loss plan if your dog is overweight.

Regular Exercise: Encourage regular physical activity, which can help improve insulin sensitivity and promote weight loss. Tailor the exercise plan to your dog's abilities and preferences.

C. Monitoring and Behavior

Regular Veterinary Check-Ups: Schedule routine visits with your veterinarian to monitor your dog's condition and make necessary adjustments to the treatment plan.

Home Monitoring: Track your dog's blood glucose levels, symptoms, and behavior. This information can help you and your veterinarian make informed decisions about your dog's care.

Note

Chapter 05

Making Treatment Decisions for Your Dog

When managing canine diabetes, making informed treatment decisions is crucial for your dog's health and well-being. Collaboration with your veterinarian and understanding your dog's lifestyle are essential components of effective management.

WORKING WITH YOUR VETERINARIAN
Collaboration with your veterinarian is vital in developing and maintaining an effective treatment plan for your diabetic dog. Here are key considerations when working with your veterinary team:

A. Open Communication
Regular Check-Ups: Schedule routine appointments to monitor your dog's condition. Frequent check-ups allow your veterinarian to assess treatment effectiveness and make necessary adjustments based on your dog's health and blood glucose levels.

Share Observations: Keep your veterinarian informed about any changes in your dog's behavior, appetite, energy levels, or any symptoms you notice. This information can help your veterinarian make informed decisions regarding treatment adjustments.

Ask Questions: Don't hesitate to ask your veterinarian questions about your dog's diabetes, treatment options, and any concerns you may have. Understanding the condition and its management can empower you to make better decisions for your dog's care.

B. Personalized Treatment Plans

Tailored Approach: Every dog is different, and treatment plans should be personalized based on your dog's specific needs, lifestyle, and health status. Your veterinarian will consider factors such as age, weight, breed, and any other health conditions when developing a treatment plan.

Insulin Management: If your dog requires insulin therapy, your veterinarian will guide you on the appropriate type of insulin, dosage, and administration techniques. They will also help you determine the best times to monitor blood glucose levels.

Dietary Recommendations: Your veterinarian can provide guidance on selecting the best diet for your dog's diabetes management. This may include specialized diabetic food or recommendations for home-cooked meals that meet your dog's nutritional needs.

C. Emergency Protocols

Recognizing Emergencies: Work with your veterinarian to understand the signs of hypoglycemia and hyperglycemia and what to do in case of an emergency. Having a clear action plan can help you respond quickly to any critical situation.

Emergency Contact Information: Keep your veterinarian's contact information handy, including after-hours emergency contacts for immediate support in case of urgent situations.

BALANCING LIFESTYLE AND TREATMENT

Balancing your dog's lifestyle with their diabetes treatment is essential for effective management. Consider the following aspects to ensure that your dog leads a fulfilling life while receiving the necessary care:

A. Dietary Modifications

Healthy Treats: Offer healthy, low-calorie treats that are appropriate for diabetic dogs. Avoid high-sugar or high-carb treats, and opt for options that support blood glucose regulation.

Home-Cooked Meals: If you prefer to prepare your dog's food at home, consult your veterinarian for guidance on creating balanced meals that meet your dog's nutritional needs while managing their diabetes.

B. Monitoring Changes

Observe Behavior: Pay close attention to your dog's behavior and well-being. Changes in appetite, energy levels, or urination can signal adjustments in their diabetes management plan may be needed.

Track Blood Glucose Levels: Regularly monitor your dog's blood glucose levels and keep a record of the readings. This data will help you identify trends and discuss them with your veterinarian during check-ups.

C. Adapting to Lifestyle Changes

Travel Considerations: If you plan to travel with your dog, make sure to bring all necessary supplies, including insulin, syringes, and any special food. Research pet-friendly accommodations and ensure your dog's routine can be maintained as much as possible.

Social Activities: Find ways to involve your diabetic dog in family activities while ensuring their dietary and exercise needs are met. Modify games or outings to suit your dog's energy levels and health status.

Note

Chapter 06

Managing Side Effects of Diabetes Treatment

Managing diabetes in dogs involves not only implementing treatment strategies but also addressing potential side effects that may arise from those treatments. Understanding these side effects, including insulin reactions and long-term complications, is crucial for ensuring your dog's health and well-being.

1. Insulin Reactions (Hypoglycemia)

Hypoglycemia, or low blood sugar, is a common side effect of insulin therapy in dogs. It can occur if your dog receives too much insulin relative to their food intake or activity level. Recognizing the signs and knowing how to respond can help prevent serious complications.

Signs of Hypoglycemia

Behavioral Changes: Look for signs such as lethargy, weakness, or confusion. Your dog may seem disoriented or have difficulty walking.

Physical Symptoms: Symptoms may include trembling, shaking, or seizures. Some dogs may also exhibit increased heart rate or panting.

Loss of Consciousness: In severe cases, hypoglycemia can lead to loss of consciousness or seizures, which require immediate veterinary attention.

Immediate Response to Hypoglycemia

If you suspect your dog is experiencing hypoglycemia, act quickly:

i. Administer Quick Sugar: Offer a source of sugar immediately, such as honey, corn syrup, or glucose gel. Rub it on your dog's gums or feed it directly, as this can quickly raise blood sugar levels.

ii. Recheck Blood Sugar Levels: If you have a glucose meter, retest your dog's blood sugar after 15-20 minutes to see if levels have returned to normal. If you don't have a meter, monitor your dog's symptoms and their responsiveness.

iii. Veterinary Consultation: After addressing the immediate situation, contact your veterinarian to discuss the incident. They may recommend adjustments to your dog's insulin dosage or feeding routine to prevent future occurrences.

Prevention of Hypoglycemia

Consistent Insulin Administration: Administer insulin at the same times each day, ensuring the dosage is appropriate for your dog's needs.

Monitor Food Intake: Ensure that your dog consumes their prescribed diet and does not skip meals. Adjust insulin doses as necessary if there are changes in appetite or feeding schedules.

Regular Monitoring: Regularly check blood glucose levels, especially during times of stress, illness, or changes in routine. This proactive approach can help identify potential issues before they escalate.

2. Long-term Complications and Prevention

While effective diabetes management can significantly improve your dog's quality of life, untreated or poorly managed diabetes can lead to long-term complications.

Common Long-term Complications

Diabetic Ketoacidosis (DKA): This serious condition occurs when the body begins to break down fat for energy instead of glucose, leading to the buildup of ketones in the blood. DKA is a medical emergency requiring immediate veterinary care.

Urinary Tract Infections (UTIs): Diabetic dogs are more susceptible to UTIs due to increased glucose in the urine, creating an environment conducive to bacterial growth. Frequent urination can also lead to dehydration.

Cataracts: Dogs with diabetes are at higher risk for developing cataracts, which can lead to vision impairment or blindness if not managed properly.

Neuropathy: Diabetes can cause nerve damage, resulting in weakness, decreased coordination, and difficulty walking. This condition can impact your dog's mobility and quality of life.

Pancreatitis: Chronic high blood sugar can lead to inflammation of the pancreas, known as pancreatitis, which can cause severe abdominal pain and other gastrointestinal issues.

Preventing Long-term Complications

Regular Veterinary Check-Ups: Schedule routine examinations and blood tests to monitor your dog's diabetes management and overall health. Early detection of complications is key to effective intervention.

Maintain Stable Blood Sugar Levels: Work closely with your veterinarian to ensure stable blood glucose levels through proper insulin administration, dietary management, and lifestyle adjustments.

Promptly Address Health Issues: Be vigilant for any signs of illness or changes in behavior. Promptly address any health concerns with your veterinarian to prevent complications from escalating.

Lifestyle Modifications: Incorporate a balanced diet and regular exercise into your dog's routine to promote weight management and overall health. Reducing stress and providing a stable environment can also positively impact your dog's well-being.

Note

Chapter 07

Nutrition and Diet for Dogs with Diabetes

Proper nutrition is a cornerstone of managing diabetes in dogs. A well-balanced diet can help regulate blood sugar levels, maintain a healthy weight, and prevent complications associated with diabetes.

Key Dietary Components

Carbohydrates: Carbohydrates have the most significant impact on blood sugar levels. High-glycemic foods can cause rapid spikes in blood glucose, while low-glycemic foods result in slower, more stable increases. Selecting high-fiber carbohydrates can help slow digestion and glucose absorption, promoting better blood sugar control.

Proteins: Adequate protein is vital for maintaining muscle mass and overall health. A diet rich in quality protein can support your dog's metabolic processes and help maintain stable blood sugar levels. Lean meats, fish, and some plant-based proteins are excellent choices.

Fats: Healthy fats are essential for overall health, providing a concentrated source of energy and aiding in nutrient absorption. Incorporate sources of omega-3 and omega-6 fatty acids, which can help reduce inflammation and support heart health.

Impact of Diet on Blood Sugar Control

Regulating Blood Glucose Levels: A balanced diet can help stabilize blood sugar levels and prevent extreme fluctuations. A consistent feeding schedule and controlled portion sizes are crucial in managing your dog's insulin response.

Weight Management: Overweight dogs are more prone to insulin resistance, making diabetes management more challenging. A diet designed for weight loss or maintenance can help your dog achieve and maintain a healthy weight, enhancing their overall metabolic health.

Before making any dietary changes, consult your veterinarian to ensure that the selected diet meets your dog's specific needs. They can help determine the appropriate caloric intake, nutrient balance, and any necessary dietary modifications based on your dog's health status.

Choosing the Right Food for Your Dog

Selecting the right food for a diabetic dog involves careful consideration of ingredients, formulation, and your dog's unique health needs. Here are some guidelines to help you make informed choices:

A. Types of Dog Food

Commercial Diabetic Diets: Many pet food manufacturers offer specialized diets formulated for diabetic dogs. These diets typically contain controlled levels of carbohydrates, higher fiber content, and balanced protein sources. Look for products labeled as "diabetic" or "weight management" that are approved by veterinarians.

Prescription Diets: Your veterinarian may recommend prescription diets specifically designed for diabetic management. These diets undergo rigorous testing to ensure they provide the right balance of nutrients for managing diabetes.

Homemade Diets: If you prefer to prepare food at home, work closely with your veterinarian to develop a balanced meal plan. Homemade diets can be tailored to meet your dog's specific needs but require careful planning to ensure they provide all essential nutrients.

B. Reading Labels

When choosing commercial dog food, carefully read the labels to understand the ingredients and nutritional content:

Ingredient Quality: Look for high-quality, identifiable ingredients. Whole meats, whole grains, and vegetables should be primary ingredients. Avoid foods with fillers, artificial additives, and high-glycemic ingredients such as corn syrup or excessive grains.

Nutritional Balance: Ensure the food meets the nutritional guidelines set by the Association of American Feed Control Officials (AAFCO), or that of your country as the case may be, for complete and balanced nutrition. This ensures your dog receives adequate nutrients to support their health.

Fiber Content: Choose foods with higher fiber content, as fiber can help regulate blood sugar levels. Ingredients like beet pulp, pumpkin, and whole grains are good sources of dietary fiber.

C. Monitoring and Adjusting Diet

Observe Your Dog's Response: After introducing a new diet, monitor your dog's blood glucose levels, weight, and overall health. Note any changes in behavior, appetite, or weight.

Be Prepared to Adjust: If you notice fluctuations in blood sugar levels or any health concerns, consult your veterinarian to reassess the diet. Adjustments may be necessary based on your dog's response to the new food.

Note

Chapter 08

Dietary Recommendations for Diabetic Dogs

Feeding a diabetic dog requires careful attention to portion sizes, meal frequency, and nutrient composition. Proper dietary management can significantly impact your dog's blood glucose levels and overall health.

Managing portion sizes and meal frequency is essential for maintaining stable blood glucose levels in diabetic dogs. Here are key considerations for portion control and feeding schedules:

Portion Control
Measure Food Accurately: Use a measuring cup or scale to ensure you are providing the correct amount of food for your dog's size, weight, and activity level. Avoid free-feeding, as this can lead to overeating and unstable blood sugar levels.

Follow Caloric Guidelines: Work with your veterinarian to determine the appropriate caloric intake for your dog. This will depend on factors such as age, weight, activity level, and overall health.

Adjust Portions as Needed: Regularly assess your dog's weight and condition. If your dog is gaining or losing weight unexpectedly, adjust portion sizes accordingly.

Meal Frequency

Consistent Feeding Schedule: Establish a consistent feeding routine by feeding your dog at the same times each day. This consistency helps regulate insulin levels and supports stable blood glucose levels.

Divide Daily Food Intake: Depending on your dog's needs, consider dividing their daily food intake into two or three smaller meals. Smaller, more frequent meals can help minimize blood sugar spikes and provide a steady source of energy.

Timing with Insulin Administration: If your dog is on insulin therapy, coordinate meal times with insulin administration as advised by your veterinarian. Administer insulin approximately 30 minutes before meals to help manage blood glucose levels effectively.

When managing a diabetic dog's diet, focusing on specific nutrients is crucial for promoting stable blood sugar levels and overall health. Here are essential nutrients to consider:

High-Quality Proteins

- ➤ ***Lean Proteins:*** Include high-quality sources of protein, such as chicken, turkey, fish, and lean cuts of beef. Protein helps maintain muscle mass, supports metabolism, and provides a sense of fullness without causing significant increases in blood sugar.
- ➤ ***Increased Protein for Weight Loss:*** If your dog is overweight, a higher protein diet can aid in weight loss while promoting lean muscle retention.

Fiber

- ➤ ***Soluble Fiber:*** Incorporate sources of soluble fiber, such as oats, barley, and legumes. Soluble fiber can slow down digestion and glucose absorption, leading to more stable blood sugar levels.
- ➤ ***Insoluble Fiber:*** Sources like pumpkin and green beans can also help with satiety and digestive health. High-fiber diets are particularly beneficial for diabetic dogs to regulate blood glucose.

Healthy Fats
- ➤ ***Omega-3 Fatty Acids:*** Include sources of omega-3 fatty acids, such as fish oil or flaxseed oil. Omega-3s have anti-inflammatory properties and may help improve insulin sensitivity.
- ➤ ***Controlled Fat Intake:*** While healthy fats are beneficial, it's important to monitor the total fat intake, especially if your dog is overweight. A balanced approach ensures that your dog receives essential fatty acids without excessive calories.

Low-Glycemic Carbohydrates
- ➤ ***Complex Carbohydrates:*** Choose low-glycemic, complex carbohydrates that provide slow-releasing energy, such as sweet potatoes, quinoa, and whole grains. These help prevent sudden spikes in blood glucose levels.
- ➤ ***Avoid Simple Sugars:*** Steer clear of foods containing simple sugars and high-glycemic ingredients, such as corn syrup, sugar, or highly processed grains. These can lead to rapid increases in blood sugar.

Chapter 09

Recipes for Diabetic Dogs

Recipe 1: Chicken and Vegetable Stew

Ingredients:
- 1 pound boneless, skinless chicken breast, diced
- 2 cups low-sodium chicken broth
- 1 cup green beans, chopped
- 1 cup carrots, diced
- 1 cup zucchini, diced
- 1/2 cup pumpkin puree (unsweetened)
- 1 tablespoon olive oil
- 1 teaspoon dried parsley

Instructions:

1. In a large pot, heat olive oil over medium heat. Add the diced chicken and cook until browned.
2. Pour in the chicken broth and bring to a simmer.
3. Add the green beans, carrots, and zucchini. Cook for about 15-20 minutes until the vegetables are tender.
4. Stir in the pumpkin puree and dried parsley. Cook for an additional 5 minutes.
5. Allow the stew to cool before serving. Store leftovers in an airtight container in the refrigerator for up to three days.

Recipe 2: Beef and Quinoa Bowl

Ingredients:
- 1 pound lean ground beef
- 1 cup quinoa, rinsed
- 2 cups water
- 1 cup spinach, chopped
- 1/2 cup carrots, grated
- 1/2 cup peas (fresh or frozen)
- 1 tablespoon fish oil (optional)

Instructions:

1. In a medium saucepan, bring water to a boil. Add quinoa, reduce heat to low, cover, and simmer for about 15 minutes until quinoa is fluffy.
2. In a skillet, brown the ground beef over medium heat until fully cooked. Drain excess fat.
3. Add spinach, carrots, and peas to the beef, and cook for another 5 minutes until vegetables are tender.
4. Mix the quinoa into the beef and vegetable mixture. If using fish oil, stir it in at this point.
5. Allow the mixture to cool before serving. Store leftovers in the refrigerator for up to three days.

Recipe 3: Turkey & Pumpkin Stew

Ingredients:

- 1 lb lean ground turkey
- 1 cup pumpkin puree (unsweetened)
- 1 cup green beans, chopped
- 1 cup cauliflower, chopped
- 1 tbsp coconut oil

Instructions:

1. Sauté turkey in a pan with coconut oil until fully cooked.
2. Add pumpkin, green beans, and cauliflower. Mix well.
3. Cook on low heat for 10-15 minutes until veggies are tender.
4. Cool before serving. Portion according to dog's size.

Recipe 4: Chicken & Spinach Bowl

Ingredients:

- 1 lb boneless, skinless chicken breast, cubed
- 1 cup spinach, chopped
- 1 cup carrots, chopped
- 1 cup zucchini, chopped
- 1 tbsp olive oil

Instructions:

1. Sauté chicken in olive oil until fully cooked.
2. Add spinach, carrots, and zucchini, stirring until veggies are tender.
3. Let cool before serving.

Recipe 5: Beef & Broccoli Delight

Ingredients:

- 1 lb lean ground beef
- 1 cup broccoli florets, chopped
- 1 cup cauliflower rice
- 1/2 cup grated carrot
- 1 tbsp flaxseed oil

Instructions:

1. Brown the beef in a pan, drain excess fat.
2. Add broccoli, cauliflower rice, and carrots; cook until tender.
3. Drizzle flaxseed oil, stir, and allow to cool before serving.

Recipe 6: Salmon & Veggie Mix

Ingredients:

- 1 lb salmon, skinless and boneless
- 1 cup spinach, chopped
- 1 cup green beans, chopped
- 1/2 cup blueberries
- 1 tbsp coconut oil

Instructions:

1. Cook salmon in coconut oil until flaky.
2. Add spinach and green beans, cooking until tender.
3. Remove from heat and mix in blueberries.
4. Let cool before feeding.

Recipe 7: Lentil & Turkey Power Bowl

Ingredients:

- 1 lb ground turkey
- 1 cup cooked lentils (unsalted)
- 1 cup carrots, chopped
- 1 cup celery, chopped
- 1 tbsp olive oil

Instructions:

1. Brown turkey in olive oil.
2. Add carrots and celery, cook until softened.
3. Stir in lentils and let cool before serving.

Recipe 8: Cottage Cheese & Spinach Mix

Ingredients:
- 1 cup low-fat cottage cheese
- 1 cup spinach, chopped
- 1 cup green beans, chopped
- 1/2 cup pumpkin puree

Instructions:
1. Steam spinach and green beans until tender, then drain.
2. Mix with cottage cheese and pumpkin.
3. Serve at room temperature.

Recipe 9: Chicken & Butternut Squash Medley

Ingredients:
- 1 lb chicken breast, cubed
- 1 cup butternut squash, cubed
- 1 cup broccoli, chopped
- 1 tbsp olive oil

Instructions:
1. Sauté chicken in olive oil until fully cooked.
2. Add butternut squash and broccoli, cook until tender.
3. Allow to cool before serving.

Recipe 10: Egg & Veggie Breakfast Scramble

Ingredients:
- 2 eggs
- 1/2 cup spinach, chopped
- 1/2 cup zucchini, grated
- 1 tbsp coconut oil

Instructions:
1. Whisk eggs, then cook in coconut oil on medium heat.
2. Add spinach and zucchini, scramble until fully cooked.
3. Cool before serving.

Recipe 11: Beef & Sweet Potato Stew

Ingredients:
- 1 lb lean ground beef
- 1 cup sweet potatoes, cubed
- 1 cup green beans, chopped
- 1 tbsp olive oil

Instructions:
1. Brown beef in a pot with olive oil.
2. Add sweet potatoes and green beans, cover with water and simmer until tender.
3. Cool and serve.

Recipe 12: Chicken & Kale Feast

Ingredients:
- 1 lb chicken breast, cubed
- 1 cup kale, chopped
- 1 cup broccoli, chopped
- 1 tbsp olive oil

Instructions:
1. Sauté chicken in olive oil until fully cooked.
2. Add kale and broccoli, cooking until tender.
3. Cool before serving.

Each of these recipes offers a balanced mix of proteins, low-glycemic veggies, and healthy fats. Be sure to store leftovers in the fridge and reheat gently, ensuring the meal is not too hot before serving.

TREATS AND SNACKS FOR DIABETIC DOGS

Recipe 1: Sweet Potato Chews

Ingredients:
- 2 medium sweet potatoes

Instructions:
1. Preheat your oven to 250°F (120°C).
2. Wash and peel the sweet potatoes. Cut them into thin slices or long strips.
3. Arrange the slices on a baking sheet lined with parchment paper.
4. Bake for about 2-3 hours, flipping halfway through, until they are dried and chewy.
5. Allow to cool completely before serving. Store in an airtight container for up to one week.

Recipe 2: Apple and Peanut Butter Treats

Ingredients:
- 1 cup whole wheat flour (or a grain-free alternative)
- 1/2 cup unsweetened applesauce
- 1/4 cup natural peanut butter (make sure it doesn't contain xylitol)
- 1 egg

Instructions:

1. Preheat your oven to 350°F (175°C).
2. In a mixing bowl, combine the flour, applesauce, peanut butter, and egg. Mix until a dough forms.
3. Roll out the dough on a floured surface to about 1/4 inch thick. Use cookie cutters to shape the treats.
4. Place the treats on a baking sheet lined with parchment paper.
5. Bake for 20-25 minutes, or until golden brown. Allow to cool completely before serving.
6. Store in an airtight container for up to one week.

Recipe 3: Apple & Carrot Bites

Ingredients:

- 1/2 cup unsweetened applesauce
- 1/2 cup grated carrots
- 1 cup oat flour
- 1 egg

Instructions:

1. Preheat the oven to 350°F (175°C).
2. Mix all ingredients in a bowl.
3. Drop small spoonfuls on a baking sheet lined with parchment paper.
4. Bake for 15-20 minutes until golden.
5. Cool completely before serving.

Recipe 4: Pumpkin & Coconut Balls

Ingredients:

- 1 cup pumpkin puree (unsweetened)
- 1/4 cup unsweetened shredded coconut
- 1/2 cup ground flaxseed

Instructions:

1. Mix pumpkin, coconut, and flaxseed in a bowl until combined.
2. Roll into small bite-sized balls.
3. Refrigerate for 1 hour before serving.

Recipe 5: Frozen Yogurt Blueberry Bites

Ingredients:

- 1 cup plain, unsweetened Greek yogurt
- 1/2 cup blueberries (fresh or frozen)

Instructions:

1. Drop small spoonfuls of yogurt on a parchment-lined tray.
2. Place a blueberry in the center of each spoonful.
3. Freeze for at least 2 hours.
4. Serve as a cool treat.

Recipe 6: Chicken Jerky Strips

Ingredients:

- 1 lb boneless, skinless chicken breast

Instructions:

1. Preheat the oven to 200°F (95°C).
2. Slice chicken into thin strips.
3. Place on a baking sheet lined with parchment paper.
4. Bake for 2-3 hours until dry and chewy.
5. Store in an airtight container and use within a week.

Recipe 7: Cucumber & Peanut Butter Bites

Ingredients:

- 1 cucumber, sliced into rounds
- 1/4 cup natural, unsweetened peanut butter

Instructions:

1. Spread a small amount of peanut butter on each cucumber slice.
2. Serve immediately as a refreshing snack.

Recipe 8: Egg & Parsley Mini Muffins

Ingredients:

- 2 eggs
- 1/4 cup chopped parsley
- 1/2 cup oat flour

Instructions:
1. Preheat the oven to 350°F (175°C).
2. Whisk eggs and add parsley and oat flour.
3. Pour mixture into mini muffin tins.
4. Bake for 10-12 minutes until set.
5. Cool before serving.

Recipe 9: Carrot & Flaxseed Crunchies

Ingredients:
- 1/2 cup grated carrot
- 1/2 cup ground flaxseed
- 1 egg

Instructions:
1. Preheat the oven to 350°F (175°C).
2. Mix all ingredients in a bowl.
3. Shape into small discs and place on a baking sheet.
4. Bake for 15 minutes until crisp.
5. Cool completely before serving.

Recipe 10: Pumpkin & Cinnamon Paws

Ingredients:
- 1/2 cup pumpkin puree (unsweetened)
- 1 egg
- 1/4 tsp cinnamon

Instructions:

1. Preheat the oven to 350°F (175°C).
2. Mix all ingredients in a bowl.
3. Drop spoonfuls on a lined baking sheet.
4. Bake for 15 minutes until firm.
5. Cool before serving.

Recipe 11: Zucchini & Parmesan Chips

Ingredients:

- 1 zucchini, thinly sliced
- 1 tbsp grated Parmesan (optional)

Instructions:

1. Preheat the oven to 250°F (120°C).
2. Place zucchini slices on a parchment-lined baking sheet.
3. Sprinkle a tiny bit of Parmesan (if desired).
4. Bake for 2 hours until crispy, flipping halfway.
5. Cool before serving.

Chapter 10

Additional Tips for Managing Diabetes in Dogs

Managing diabetes in dogs requires a comprehensive approach that goes beyond diet and medication. Regular exercise and diligent monitoring of blood glucose levels play critical roles in ensuring your dog's health and well-being.

REGULAR EXERCISE AND ACTIVITY

Physical activity is essential for all dogs, but it is especially important for diabetic dogs. Regular exercise helps regulate blood sugar levels, maintain a healthy weight, and promote overall health. Some of the benefits of exercise are;

Blood Sugar Control: Exercise can help lower blood glucose levels by increasing insulin sensitivity and facilitating glucose uptake by the muscles. This helps prevent spikes in blood sugar after meals.

Weight Management: Regular physical activity helps maintain a healthy weight, reducing the risk of insulin resistance. Weight loss can significantly improve diabetes management in overweight dogs.

Mental Stimulation: Exercise provides mental engagement, reducing boredom and anxiety. A mentally stimulated dog is generally happier and more content.

Types of Exercise

- *Walking:* Daily walks are a great way to ensure your dog gets the exercise they need. Aim for at least 30 minutes of walking each day, divided into two sessions if needed.
- *Playtime:* Interactive play, such as fetch or tug-of-war, can be an enjoyable way to engage your dog physically and mentally.
- *Swimming:* If your dog enjoys water, swimming can be an excellent low-impact exercise option that helps build strength and endurance without putting stress on the joints.

Tips for Exercise

Consistency is Key: Establish a regular exercise routine to help regulate your dog's blood sugar levels. Aim for the same duration and intensity of exercise each day.

Monitor Intensity: Be mindful of your dog's energy levels and adjust the intensity of the exercise as needed. Avoid strenuous activities if your dog is not accustomed to them, especially if they have been inactive for a while.

Post-Exercise Monitoring: After exercise, monitor your dog's blood glucose levels, as they may experience a drop. This is especially important if you've recently adjusted their insulin dosage or diet.

Also paramount is the regular monitoring of blood glucose levels which is crucial for effective diabetes management in dogs. It allows you to make informed decisions about diet, exercise, and insulin administration. Here's how to implement routine monitoring effectively:

Home Testing: Familiarize yourself with home glucose monitoring techniques. Your veterinarian can guide you on how to use a glucometer, which is a device that measures blood sugar levels.

Frequency of Testing: Work with your veterinarian to establish how often you should test your dog's blood glucose levels. This may vary based on your dog's condition, medication, and treatment plan, but a common practice is to test before meals and insulin administration.

Interpreting Blood Glucose Levels

Normal Range: Understand what constitutes a normal blood glucose range for your dog. Generally, a blood glucose level of 80-120 mg/dL is considered normal, but your veterinarian will provide specific target ranges based on your dog's individual needs.

Signs of High and Low Blood Sugar: Learn to recognize signs of hyperglycemia (high blood sugar) and hypoglycemia (low blood sugar). Common signs include increased thirst and urination, lethargy, and loss of appetite for hyperglycemia; trembling, weakness, confusion, and seizures for hypoglycemia.

Chapter 11

Alternative Therapies for Canine Diabetes

In addition to traditional medical treatments, various alternative therapies can complement diabetes management in dogs. These therapies can help support overall health, enhance well-being, and address specific needs associated with diabetes.

1. Herbal and Natural Supplements
Herbal and natural supplements can provide additional support for diabetic dogs, potentially aiding in blood sugar regulation and promoting overall health. However, it's crucial to consult with your veterinarian before introducing any supplements to ensure they are safe and appropriate for your dog's specific condition.

A. Common Herbal and Natural Supplements
Cinnamon: This spice is believed to help improve insulin sensitivity and lower blood sugar levels. Cinnamon can be added in small amounts to your dog's food.

Bitter Melon: This plant has been traditionally used to help regulate blood sugar levels. Bitter melon can be found in supplement form or as a powder to mix into your dog's food.

Berberine: Derived from several plants, berberine has been studied for its potential to lower blood sugar levels and improve insulin sensitivity. It is available in supplement form.

Omega-3 Fatty Acids: Supplements like fish oil or flaxseed oil can provide omega-3 fatty acids, which may help reduce inflammation and improve overall metabolic health. These can be beneficial for diabetic dogs, particularly if they are overweight.

Alpha-Lipoic Acid (ALA): This antioxidant may help improve insulin sensitivity and support overall metabolic health. It is available in supplement form.

B. Considerations for Using Supplements

Consult Your Veterinarian: Always discuss any herbal or natural supplements with your veterinarian before giving them to your dog. Some supplements may interact with medications or may not be appropriate for dogs with certain health conditions.

Quality of Supplements: Choose high-quality, reputable brands when selecting supplements. Look for those that have been tested for safety and efficacy.

Monitor Your Dog's Response: Keep an eye on your dog for any changes in behavior, appetite, or health after introducing a new supplement. Report any concerns to your veterinarian.

2. Acupuncture and Other Complementary Treatments

Acupuncture and other complementary therapies can provide additional support for managing diabetes in dogs. These treatments can help alleviate symptoms, reduce stress, and promote overall well-being.

A. Acupuncture

How It Works: Acupuncture involves inserting thin needles into specific points on the body to stimulate energy flow and promote healing. It can help improve blood circulation, relieve pain, and support overall health.

Benefits for Diabetic Dogs: Acupuncture may help regulate blood sugar levels, improve insulin sensitivity, and reduce the side effects of diabetes. It can also alleviate stress and anxiety, which can positively impact diabetes management.

Finding a Qualified Practitioner: Look for a veterinarian trained in veterinary acupuncture. They will assess your dog's condition and create a tailored treatment plan.

B. Other Complementary Therapies

Massage Therapy: Therapeutic massage can help improve circulation, reduce stress, and promote relaxation. It may be beneficial for diabetic dogs to support overall well-being and muscle health.

Physical Therapy: For diabetic dogs, especially those that are overweight or have mobility issues, physical therapy can help improve strength, flexibility, and overall fitness. A physical therapist can develop a customized exercise plan.

Chiropractic Care: Chiropractic adjustments can help ensure proper spinal alignment, which may improve nerve function and overall health. Some dogs with diabetes may benefit from chiropractic care as part of a comprehensive management plan.

Homeopathy: Some dog owners explore homeopathic remedies to support their dog's health. Consult with a veterinarian trained in homeopathy to ensure safe and appropriate treatment options.

Note

Chapter 12

Emotional Support for You and Your Family

Managing a dog's diabetes can take an emotional toll on both you and your family. It is vital to recognize and address the emotional impact of this diagnosis, as well as to find effective ways to support your dog's health and happiness.

Coping with Your Dog's Diagnosis
Receiving a diagnosis of diabetes for your dog can be overwhelming. It is natural to experience a mix of emotions, including fear, sadness, and uncertainty about the future. Understanding how to cope with these feelings can make the journey easier for both you and your dog.

A. Acknowledge Your Emotions

Recognize Your Feelings: It is important to allow yourself to feel whatever emotions arise. This might include sadness over your dog's health, anxiety about treatment, or frustration with managing their condition.

Accept That It's Okay to Feel Sad: Understand that grieving the loss of your dog's previous health is part of the process. Embrace these feelings rather than suppress them.

B. Educate Yourself

Gather Information: Knowledge is empowering. Learn as much as you can about canine diabetes, its management, and treatment options. This can alleviate some of your fears and help you feel more in control.

Consult with Your Veterinarian: Establishing a strong relationship with your veterinarian can provide guidance and reassurance. They can answer questions and help you understand what to expect moving forward.

C. Build a Support Network

Lean on Family and Friends: Share your feelings and concerns with family members or close friends who understand your situation. Emotional support can be invaluable during this time.

Join Support Groups: Connecting with other pet owners facing similar challenges can provide comfort and practical advice. Look for local or online support groups for pet diabetes.

D. Focus on Self-Care

Prioritize Your Well-being: Caring for a diabetic dog can be demanding, so it's essential to take care of yourself. Ensure you're getting enough rest, eating well, and finding time for activities you enjoy.

Practice Stress-Relief Techniques: Engage in mindfulness practices, such as meditation or yoga, to help manage stress and maintain a positive mindset.

Supporting Your Dog's Well-being

Your dog's emotional and physical well-being is crucial for effective diabetes management. Providing them with love, care, and comfort can make a significant difference in their quality of life.

A. Establish a Routine

Consistency is Key: Dogs thrive on routine. Establish regular feeding, exercise, and insulin administration times to create stability in your dog's life. This can also help regulate their blood sugar levels.

Predictable Environment: Keep their environment consistent and free from drastic changes to minimize stress.

B. Offer Emotional Comfort

Show Affection: Physical touch, such as petting or cuddling, can provide emotional support and reassurance to your dog. Your calm presence can help alleviate their anxiety.

Quality Time Together: Spend time engaging in activities your dog enjoys, such as gentle play or leisurely walks. This fosters a sense of normalcy and happiness.

C. Monitor Their Behavior and Health

Watch for Changes: Be attentive to your dog's mood and behavior. Changes in appetite, energy levels, or general demeanor can indicate issues that may need veterinary attention.

Keep a Health Journal: Document any changes in your dog's condition, including blood sugar levels, eating habits, and behavior. This record can be useful for discussions with your veterinarian.

D. Regular Veterinary Check-ups

Schedule Routine Appointments: Regular check-ups are essential for managing your dog's diabetes. These visits help track progress, adjust treatments, and catch any potential complications early.

Open Communication: Maintain an open line of communication with your veterinarian. Share any concerns and discuss your dog's health and treatment progress.

Note

Conclusion

The journey of managing canine diabetes can be overwhelming at times, but it is also an opportunity to strengthen the bond you share with your dog. Your dedication to their care can lead to improved health and a longer, happier life together. Remember that you are not alone, many resources, support groups, and veterinary professionals are available to help you navigate this path.

With compassion, patience, and proactive care, you can ensure your beloved pet thrives despite their diabetes. Embrace the journey, and take pride in the care and love you provide as you work together to manage their condition. Your commitment will make all the difference in your dog's life, allowing them to enjoy every moment by your side.

www.ingramcontent.com/pod-product-compliance
Lightning Source LLC
Chambersburg PA
CBHW071054240526
45469CB00006BD/2299